MASSAGE – RUB A DUB DUB

Theresa Hollis

Books by the same author

The Sabbath

Names have been changed to protect the innocent!

To all my clients who survived!
Thank You

CHAPTER ONE

I live in a small country town in New South Wales (that's Australia for those that are trying to find it on a world map).

It is a town where everyone knows everyone else or is related to them, which makes for an interesting time if you forget and mention that so and so did this or that, which I have tended to do on more than one occasion, only to be told that that is their aunt, cousin or brother. Talk about foot in mouth, fortunately most people see the funny side of things and then proceed to tell you stories of said person, some of which would make your hair curl.

The joys of living in small town.

It does have its good points though, everybody knows who you are and says hello. The down side is being a divorced women AND a Massage Therapist everyone knows, or thinks they know, things about you that you would rather they did not.

Sometimes I think it would just be easier to put a notice in the local paper which would save an awful lot of time and bother, but then again if they are talking about me, well you know the saying they are leaving someone else alone.

Hmm not sure that is right either.

Well I like it here anyway, and working five and a half days a week from Monday to Saturday keeps me pretty well out of mischief, well most of the time.

I have Sundays off, no nothing to do with going to church, that is not my way at all as those that know me well understand. It is simply to recharge my batteries, take a swig at normality (and I have no idea what the hell that is anyway) and get ready to start the whole process all over again come Monday.

Sunday as far as I am concerned is my day off to laze and play with my dog and generally do very little.

Sounds good on paper, rarely works in real life.

Take last Sunday for instance, I had just gotten out of the shower when there was a knock on the front door.

I grab my clothes and throw them on and open the door, and yes, you guessed it, the perennial Jehovah's Witness at the door trying to save my soul.

Well guess what my soul is well past saving and if I believed in the 'Heaven/Hell thing' then Hell would have first dibs on it. So excuse me if I shoot you with silver bullets maybe that way you will get the message I am NOT interested.

Damn, now that makes another job I have to do, clean up the grey dust heaped on the front veranda, funny do not feel like brunch now.

Oh well think I will take my dog for a walk, so I grab his lead with the harness attached then try and calm him down so that I can put the damned thing on.

When exactly was the last time I took him for a walk? Finally after a great deal of contortion work on my part and great patience on his I get the harness on.

We head off out the door and chuff off down the road deciding that we might as well do some window shopping on the way and maybe stop at the local bakery and get a coffee for my dog and a bun for me, no hang on there is something wrong there!

Well we make it to the bakery, but only after every tree, stick, fence, bin and blade of grass has been adequately christened by my dog.

What you thought it was me? Please some decorum needed here folks!

Anyway now we can settle down and enjoy our rewards. Grabbing a table outside the bakery I pour some water into Jack's portable drink bowl – yes I have a Jack Russell dog and his name is Jack.

How original I hear you say, well excuse me, he is my dog and I will call him what I want, actually I never really thought about it when I named him.

I loved watching a show on television called 'Will and Grace and Will's pal was a gay guy with a wicked sense of humour who was named Jack and the name seemed right for my dog.

Gay dog? No I do not have a gay dog thank you very much it was just the name and all and you see.....oh bother it.

After our repast we decided to head off to the park and check out the pigeons, Jack is still no sure exactly what they are but boy do they move when you chase them.

No, not me chasing them, Jack chasing them what is it with you people.

Anyway after several games of pigeon chase and a walk around the park we set off back home.

Now if I am really lucky I will make it home without having a heart attack. Who said exercise is good for you should take Jack (who is convinced he is a Rottweiler in disguise) for a walk. I will guarantee that you will change your mind, talk about a team of huskies on the end of the lead, wonder how we would go in the winter Olympics at sledding, no, well just a thought.

We eventually get home in one piece, Jack heads for his water bowl and I head for the couch and collapse.

Next thing the phone rings, it is Samantha a good friend of ours she is taking her dog for a walk and do we want to come.

I tell her we have just survived a walk but if she wants to come back here later for a drink that would be great.

She says yes and to expect her in about an hour, just open the door and stick the drink on the table she is sure she will be able to manage to crawl to it by then.

Somehow I know just how she feels.

I hang up and go back to the couch, just as I am about to drift off there is a knock on the front door, again.

Who the hell is knocking on the door surely not another Jehovah's Witness it took me ages to clean up the veranda after the last lot.

Jack has run to the door, his hackles are standing on end and there is a deep growling in his throat, now that is not good.

I open the door to find my neighbor from four doors up on the doorstep.

"Hi, just wondered if you would like to go to the club tonight for a drink after tea?"

Now this neighbor has the record for not only being the biggest tight ass in town but also the worst sleaze in town.

"Gee, go for a drink after tea, how sweet of you. Now I am sure that you won't mind if my girlfriend and six of her friends come, oh then there is Max, dear Max I could not possibly go out without asking him, but that would mean that his three best mates would be coming as well, oh and I almost forgot Clive the bouncer from the Club now he really is good value for money, and......."

"Oh sorry did I say tonight, gee I forgot I umm have to work tonight, some other time then, ok, bye."

I close the door and look down at Jack who I swear is smiling at me.

"Works like a charm ever time hey boy."

I wandered into the kitchen and put the jug on to make a coffee, and then I got out a packet of chocolate teddy bear biscuits, nothing like chocolate teddies to make you feel better.

I had just finished my coffee when Jack ran to the front door, this time with tail wagging and big smile on his face. A joyful bark announced that my girlfriend must have arrived.

On opening the door there stood PeaBeu my girlfriends dog who is also a Jack Russell (see some people have excellent taste in dogs).

"Hi PeaBeu where is your boss, somewhere not far behind I bet."

Sure enough a few minutes later Samantha arrived.

"I knew you would not be far behind, PeaBeu is in the kitchen sharing some of Jack's dog biscuits and the wine for us is about to be poured." Samantha smiled, 'Halleluiah there is justice in the world, pour on."

I open a bottle of wine and put out some cheese and biscuits and we settle down to enjoy our repast and discuss relevant topics of interest. Mainly house renovation and work.

As we were drinking our wine I tell Samantha about my sleazy neighbor and his 'offer' of drinks. She laughed when I told her how I got rid of him.

"Serves him right, you would think that he would know by now that no-one wants to go out with him, creep that he is…. But I did hear that a certain married woman had been seen at his place quite a bit lately and late at night. She must really be desperate."

"Really who is she, I have not heard or seen anything, has there been anything else of interest happening around town that I don't know about?"

Samantha looked at me and laughed, "Anytime you miss something I'll dance naked down the main street at lunchtime girl!"

Well that is something that people would love to see and would cause quite a stir. Samantha is six feet tall and built like an Amazon and very striking looking.

Me, I am five foot four inches in height, cuddly best to describe my full figure and well I will never fall flat on my face if you get my meaning.

Samantha is an amazing person, she too is doing up an old house (oh did I forget to tell you that, well both of us are doing up our homes, this is the second home that I have done up, yes I know I have to be nuts).

Anyway back to Samantha, her house looks amazing she is one of those people who no matter what they tackle it always seems to be looking great, whilst I on the other hand muddle through just trying to survive on getting it right – well ok so the house I did up prior to this looked wonderful and this one is coming up trumps also.

You know working all week and most weekends and any spare time is spent on the house, life in the fast lane does have its drawbacks, there is no time for dating.

Well I suppose I did manage to fit it in a while back, there was this guy I went out with for short time. Actually I had known him for some years and sort of 'fell' into dating him that is until Valentine's Day when he got the big heave ho.

I mean how would you feel if your guy turned up on your front doorstep at 8.00pm at night with no flowers, no card, no nothing. I ask you and then he admitted that he had already had dinner thanks before he came. It is still amazing how the hell he managed to dodge the bullets I fired at him as he ran for his car.

I can laugh at it now, but at the time felt downright angry and short changed, how come everybody else gets the good guys, how about saving some of them for us who may not be quite perfect, and do not manage to look like a plastic Barbie doll 24/7 and actually like food.

Well Samantha and I discussed the pros and cons of the single male over several hours and innumerable bottles of wine.

It took a bit of mind numbing torturous hours to decide that the reason there are no eligible men in the world are: a) they are all married, b) they are all gay, c) they are living on Mars, which is why single girls the world over are standing in line to be the first on THAT spaceship.

As for me, I'm going to pilot the damned thing, I wonder if Martians are really green? My idea is that they look like a cross between Johnny Depp and Clark Gable (Oh come on you must know who Clark Gable is) no, god am I really that old.

Well by this time we are really quite merry and wander out to the back veranda which is glassed in and has been divided into two sections with wooden partitions.

"You know." Said Samantha, "This would look much better with the partitions gone."

So out to the shed we go and get a couple of hammers and then back inside we march.

We start swinging and you know what there is a lot to be said for the simple act of smashing walls down. Really someone should start up a therapy class doing this, just think of the possibilities.

Anyway an hour and a half later we have demolished the two partitions and guess what! It does look better, now all we have to do is clean up the mess, but first things first. I am starving so go and order a pizza, as we sit among the rubble waiting for the pizza we contemplate the rest of the veranda, damn so much to do and just the two of us to do it.

Ok how about we forget about it for now and open another bottle of wine, things always look better after a drink (or was that things always look better in the morning) never mind a drink it is.

CHAPTER TWO

I don't remember much of the rest of the night. I do vaguely remember crawling into bed after waving Samantha and PeaBeu off.

The next thing I remember is the clanging of bells, I managed to open one eye and see the alarm clock dancing all over the bedside cabinet. One almighty sweep sure stopped that noise, but it also means I now have to buy a new alarm clock.

Hell 7.30am already, time to get up and face the day, hopefully a shower will restore my equilibrium or at least make me feel more human. Heaven help any client who gets on the wrong side of me today.

An hour later refreshed and restored by a cup of coffee I check over the diary for Monday's bookings. I have five clients booked in from 10.00 am through to 4.30 pm, quite a busy day, time to get going and set up the clinic.

I have the clinic attached to my home which is much easier and more convenient for me (and cheaper than renting a shop).

I get the clients file notes out ready for the day ahead and make up the massage table and put the heater on to warm the room up, can't have cold clients.

My first client arrives just before 10.00 am, Maggie Dearheart who is an elderly lady who suffers from severe sciatic pain and lower back pain and has been coming to be for several years now.

I know it gives her relief from the pain and I also think that she likes to have someone to talk to, with being on her own and her only daughter living inter-state I know she gets very lonely.

Maggie gets undressed and settles herself on the massage table. As I start to work on her she tells me she has not had a good week, she 'survives' on a Age Pension and is a very independent person who wants to stay in the little house she has been renting for about the past eight years.

It seems that the landlord has decided to put the rent up which means that Maggie will find it even harder to manage (I must say that I give her a very generous discount mainly so that I can keep an eye on her and also to help ease her pain somewhat).

I do worry about her, and indeed about a lot of my elderly clients all in similar circumstances about how they will manage, but I particularly worry about Maggie.

I know that she has a cat that she adores and she tends to skimp on her own food to enable her to buy 'treats' for it. Personally I think it is the cat from hell, one mean son of a bitch that would make Attila the Hun look good, anyway she loves it and spoils it rotten, now why does that sound familiar?

I tactfully sound her out, (yes I can be tactful, well sometimes) about her situation and ask if she would not be better off moving to a cheaper place where she and Ratseemus, yes that is the name of her cat, would fare better.

She tells me that she loves it where she is as she knows all the neighbours and they all look after each other and she feels safe there.

She did confide that she is worrying about how she will manage the new rent. I suggest that maybe she could have a talk with Centerlink about her situation and see if they could help, especially with the new rental which will put her into the rate for government help.

After a bit more discussion she says that she will go and have a talk to them and see if anything can be done.

As we finish up I feel a lot better about her and make a mental note to check with her on her next visit in a fortnight's time.

As she is leaving I manage to convince her to take some eggs from my chooks (all three of them that I have running around a huge pen in the back yard).

I tell her that they have been going into mass production lately and that she would be doing me a favour to the eggs, in actual fact I think that the chooks think that it may be chicken soup time for them as I sort of mentioned that they were not producing well a couple of weeks ago and chicken soup looked good. Funny how they have excelled themselves lately, amazing things chooks and seemingly very intelligent.

On saying goodbye I look at the clock and find that I have gone over my time limit once again and will really have to get a move on to have the clinic ready for the next client.

Just as I am finishing putting clean towels on the table the bell rings and my next client is here.

This time it is a local Council worker who has managed to pull the muscles in his lower lumber, Ray Duneen who 'lumbers' into the room, and I say lumber as he is a rather – shall we say fairly corpulent man, I did NOT say fat! I look at my table and say a prayer to the 'Massage Gods' that my table will hold up.

Ray comes in chatting away as usual, I leave him to get undressed then a few minutes later return to start the massage.

Ray is sitting on the table, and yes it is still standing, and at least he got on the table this time, last time he could not move to get himself up off the chair and onto it, at least we are progressing.

I managed to get him lying on his stomach and proceed to examine his lower lumbar and his thoracic regions to see how things are progressing.

All seems to be going a lot better, and the tenderness he has been experiencing of late seem a lot better, however there are still a few spots that will need extra work.

I proceed to go to work on him. As I am massaging Ray starts to tell me all about his week at work, (he is on light duties, which seems to mean that he sits around and does some paperwork or the like) anyway it seems all is not right in Council Heaven and Ray has decided that I am the one to spill his guts to, I just hope not literally.

We has, and I use this term loosely, 'worked' for the Local Council for the past twenty years and feels that he has done enough and now it is time to 'ease off' as he puts it and make the younger guys do all the heavy lifting and the like. Especially now as he has done himself an injury whilst working above and beyond the call of duty, yes he really did say that, he then proceeds to outline all the wrongs that have been done to him over the years starting with his parents – yes that's right always blame the parents as if we have not suffered enough.

Oh I did tell you that I am also the local physiatrist did I not, at least that is what most seem to think, hmm next book could be a doozy.

Anyway back to the story, it turns out that he wants to be put on light duties permanently and was having trouble getting anywhere with his boss who just happens to be the head of the maintenance division and is supposedly a very happily married man and a keen supporter of the junior athletics, the annual pie baking contest and also helps little old ladies across the street, heaven help him if the tried to help me across any street.

Sorry I digress, to get back to what Ray was saying.

Turns out that Ray was working back later than usual one day last week and called into the general office to drop the keys to the truck back a was off on an RDO the next day and the truck was wanted for some work at the depot.

Just as Ray was putting the keys on the board he heard a noise next door, thinking it might be his mate Joe one of the cleaners, he opened the door and low and behold.

Here is Mr. Self-righteous in a state of undress – Rays' actual words were, 'kick ass naked with his bare bum in the air and his dick stuck in his Secretary.'

The said Secretary was blatantly upended on the desk with her knickers on the floor and her legs pointing towards the ceiling enjoying the workout she was getting.

Well it is funny how Ray is to now get his light duties after all and a pay rise to boot.

Of course all this was a secret between him and me, and if I know Ray, probably half the town by now, I do wonder however if Mr. Self-righteous will get nominated for Citizen of the Year this year?

After Ray left I thought back on what he had said this manager is always so prime and proper and so 'I am' – and he has a lovely wife and gorgeous young children. And the Secretary, well shall we say she has something of a 'reputation' around town and the word is that she worked her way up from a lowly filing-clerk to Secretary in a very short time and apparently all done 'on her back'.

Who said that nothing ever happens in Council.

I did hear about six months later that not only had Mr. Self-righteous' 'resigned' from his job – apparently upping the Secretary one too many times and was caught out by the General Manager late one night, the said GM having come back into the office after a meeting and finding them both in the throes of passion. Next day he and the Secretary were given their marching orders but also that his wife has tossed him out of the marital home also.

Last thing that I heard about him was that he was living somewhere in Queensland and the Secretary had taken up employment elsewhere also, but not anywhere in his vicinity.

Well the day progressed and just as I was to get ready for my last client, and glad I was, than the phone rang. It was Debbie to say that she would be running about half an hour late would it still be alright to come. Me being me said yes that would be fine.

So that gave me some time to throw some vegies together with a couple of lamb chops in the oven for tea all set on low which meant that I would have tea cooked by the time I finished the massage.

I also put all the used towels into the washing machine and did a quick tidy up of the kitchen.

Debbie arrives and apologies for being late, it appears that she had to work late as her replacement failed to turn up (Debbie is Manager of the local supermarket and has had innumerable problems with staff) I wonder could it be that she is an absolute bitch and thinks that everyone should bow down to her, not in this day and age.

Anyway I leave her to undress and going back in again shortly and start work on her.

As I am massaging her back she starts to complain that her back hurts and the massage is too firm, her right leg is numb, her neck is sore (probably from someone metaphysically trying to strangle her) she goes on to say that no-one at work understands her or the pressure she is under, all her staff are worthless etc.

She then goes on to say that her husband does not appreciate her either and he is hardly every home but spends a great deal of his time at the pub.

I can actually feel for him and understand why.

By this time she has just about run down everyone in town – I tell you what some people just beg for a hard ass massage, she is going to be a lot sorer when she gets off the table than when she got on.

Well an hour later all finished and dusted for the day it is now time for a well-earned drink, tea for both me and Jack.

As I settle down with a glass of wine I check my answering machine. There are two new appointments wanted for Wednesday and four other regulars wanting to book in, also several hang up's which is unusual. Oh well they can ring back later as the answering machine will be turned off and the phone back on to normal.

It is funny how some people hate using answering machines, I have one dear old thing who tells me, "I won't talk on those awful machines they are so inhuman."

I know there is some logic in there somewhere but I am damned if I know where.

You know it is funny but I just realized that I am on my way to being one of those funny old ladies. I can just see myself at 90 still massaging, "What did you say dear, I'm massaging your boobs, and sorry thought your knees were a bit soft and bumpy."

Maybe there is a retirement home for old massage therapists, I can just see it now.

"Slippery Arms" home for the haggard therapist, yes dear book me in now just make sure that the fridge is well stocked with booze and the phone has been ripped out of the wall and my Jack is most welcome.

Now before we go any further with this let's get one thing clear. My 'working attire' consists of knee length white shorts and a green polo necked shirt in summer and jeans in winter.

Sorry to disappoint you but I do not wear tight leather gear, like long thigh high stiletto boots and carry a whip – mind you some of the clients would love that, there is Mr......but no, that would be telling.

This is a legitimate business no 'funny stuff' here if you please, well not that sort of funny business, well just business, well, oh damn it you know what I mean.

CHAPTER THREE

Well the week goes fast and Saturday rolls around once again and I have only one client booked in. A young man who injured his knee playing football, personally why anyone would want to chase a ball around and then have someone, jump, kick, punch and generally try to annihilate you is beyond me.

Now golf is a nice sport, you hit a small ball around 18 holes and try not to hit a tree, land in the water, dodge someone else's flying ball or have a tantrum when you miss the hole and land in the long grass somewhere on the edge of the course.

Then you manage to crawl to the last hole and hit the damn ball for the last time, pick all your gear up that you may have strewn along the course as you went, then stagger into the clubhouse for a drink, now doesn't that sound more like fun.

Well before I know it my young client is here along with hid day. In they troop, this is the first time that the young man has ever been to a massage therapist, his coach referred him to me (nice man I get all his injured players, football does have its good side).

Joel Porter is just 17 and looks scared to death, his dad mentions that Joel is afraid of needles and as I use Acupuncture with my massage maybe I could not use them this time.

I explain that I do not use Acupuncture but Acupressure which is a Chinese type massage only using my finger and thumb and no needles and that he has nothing to fear.

Acupressure is all to do with certain pressure points on the body, when pressed they stimulate that part of the body to 'fix' the sore spot, the pressure is usually on for just a minute then I release it and massage over it.

I tell him that his combined with the traditional massage has wonderful results for a lot of people and stimulates the healing process, I also tell him that he will be sore after the massage and probably tired and the best thing he can do is rest for a short time after.

By this time Joel is looking more relaxed and his dad is positively beaming, "See told you son it would be ok, nothing to worry about you'll be right as rain in no time."

You know sometimes I just love parents.

Ten minutes later after completing all the relevant paper work and getting Joel settled on the table I start working on him. I always do a full body massage with new clients to make sure that there is nothing else out of place or to see if there is anything that needs special attention.

Joel starts to relax about halfway through the massage and then starts to ask questions. The usual ones, do you need much training to be a masseur – only about all of the 18 years that I have been working yes, you do need training.

You start out usually under the supervision and training of a qualified masseur who will take you through the basic training which is about 100 hours work leading up to getting your first two Certificates in Massage,

Then you can go on to do your Diploma of Massage which can be done either by correspondence or by a year full time study 'in house' and the cost is about $5000.

Once you have these there is always something new to learn and it really is an on-going training all the time.

Joel says it seems like hard work and asks the million dollar question, 'do your hands hurt?' I explain that yes it is hard work but I use my bod as well as my hands (stop jumping to conclusions by my body I mean that I center myself and take the full work load throughout my body). Then the next question, 'Do I like being a masseur?"

Now to answer that truthfully there are times when I wonder what the hell I am doing it for, then there are others when I look back at how I have helped a lot of people manage to survive from week to week and improve their way of life, then yes, I love it.

It is at this stage that his dad asks if I can do anything with sciatic pain, boy can I.

Now this is where I come into my element I tell him of the clients I have coming in for just such a complaint and describe the treatment which is a combination of massage and Chinese Acupressure and the excellent results I am getting.

Well next thing I know I have another new client booked in next week for treatment.

Told you I love football!

Just as I am cleaning up after Joel and his dad have left, the phone rings. It is a Mrs. Smyth who informs me that her son has injured himself during football training this morning and he is in a lot of pain, would he be able to come in straight away.

I tell her that I have just finished with a client and have a vacancy now (well a little white lie never hurt, no point in saying I had only the one client booked in this morning.)

I tell her to bring her son in, this was my first big mistake.

Fifteen minutes later Mrs. Smyth arrives with her son in tow. I have never seen such a sulky looking boy in all my life, if he is not careful he will fall over his bottom lip and break his neck, (which as it turned out might be a good thing).

Well in they come and Mrs. Smyth proceeds to tell me that her darling boy (second warning here) has injured his hamstring and is in sooo much pain that they just had to find someone to treat him today.

Third warning, but no, I proceed to ascertain his injury.

It turns out that not only has he pulled a hamstring but he has a nice corked muscle in his calf as well, now this is going to be fun, for me, not him.

I start to work on Winston's leg (yes that is the poor boy's name, no wonder he looks so unhappy). I gradually increase the pressure to work out the cork and alleviate the pulled hamstring, I must admit that he has not said a word or screamed so he goes up a point in my estimation.

Not so his dear mother!

"What are you doing, why is that necessary, must you cause him pain, why are you bending his leg up?"

Lady if you do not shut up you will not only get your leg bent but will find out what pain is, I don't actually say this, just think it.

I carefully explain as I work what I am doing and how it will help her dear Winston.

An hour later massage complete I advise Mrs. Smyth that her son will need a follow-up treatment next week and what day would suit.

Well here comes the punch line.

"Oh no, I will be taking Winston to his usual massage man in Wagga Wagga next week he could not fit us in today so you had to do."

Well talk about rude, I gritted my teeth took her money and just as he was leaving said.

"Well I am glad that I was able to help, by the way when you next have an emergency injury that needs attention please be so kind as to NOT contact me, I have genuine clients in need of my services and I am not and never have been a 'fill-in' for anyone. Have a nice day."

With that I show them the door and every so politely slam it, but not before I notice that Winston has turned and not only smiled at me but winked also, I could get to like that boy, pity about the mother though.

Well that is it for another week, time to clean up the clinic, wash all the towels and then just chill out for the rest of the week-end, my time is at hand.

After lunch and a bit of a rest I decided to tackle some more of the restoration awaiting me. So armed with my trust paint brush and large can of paint I proceed to tackle painting the back veranda which Samantha and I had previously renovated with a hammer and crow bar.

Several hours and three-quarters of the veranda painted I willingly clean up the brush, put the lid on the paint can and stand back and survey my handiwork.

It is amazing what a difference a coat of paint makes, the veranda is starting to look really good.

I decided to have a shower then take Jack for a walk and pick up some Chinese take-away for tea on the way home.

A short time later we head off, Jack is pleased to be going out and I am feeling refreshed and looking forward to the walk.

An hour later we arrive back home complete with take-away food, both of us very exhausted. Feed Jack then pour myself a glass of wine and open the take-away, it really is amazing how good food tastes when you don't have to cook it yourself.

I was halfway through eating when the phone rings, I glance at the clock it is after 7.00pm. I answer the phone to be greeted by, "Is this the Masseuse?"

Now if I was my usual bright self that greeting should have warned me what was to follow.

"Yes, what can I do for you?"

"I want a massage, I'm staying at the River Motel, Room 21, just knock and come in."

It is then that the warning bells go off, this is not a legitimate massage that the creep wants, ok two can play at this.

"Well let's see, I presume you want the *special* that is the hot boiling wax poured over your crown jewels and then when the wax is dry, rip it off in one excruciatingly painful go, then I gently rub a mixture of cayenne pepper and crushed chilies on you, then.......hello?"

Gee he has hung up, wonder why??

I smiled to myself it was funny now, but when I first started massaging the calls were anything but funny.

I averaged a couple a week, some were quite disgusting in their requests, one that still stands out all these years later was a guy who phoned asking if I would 'do him, whilst his mate did me', I remember being upset for weeks after that call.

It took me awhile to learn to ignore them and point out that I was a Remedial Massage Therapist who worked on torn muscles, aching backs, sciatica, injuries and the like for a living and it did not involve sex.

I must admit there were times when I would have loved to get some of them, including the guy above, on the massage table. I reckon after a session they would never bother another legitimate massage therapist ever again, probably never bother any massage person again.

I went back to my dinner, and giving Jack a pat finished it off and poured another glass of wine.

CHAPTER FOUR

The rest of the week-end past in relative peace, Samantha had gone away for a few days so my demolition buddy would not be around to help.

I decided to take things easy and just laze around and read a book and chill out. I 'chilled out' too much as next thing I knew I woke with a start to find Jack licking my face and trying to work out if I was ever going to feed him.

Heavens the day had gone in the blink of an eye. Struggling awake I rolled off the bed and stumbled into the bathroom. Washing my face and combing my hair I felt better, now to feed my erstwhile companion and myself and then see what was on TV.

On the way to the living-room I stopped off at the clinic and checked the next week's bookings. There were 22 people booked in which would make it fairly busy, plus I had no doubt that I would pick up a few more during the week.

Glancing through I saw that Melanie East was booked in for Tuesday, she was a lovely young woman with two gorgeous children aged four and seven. Melanie had survived breast cancer and was in remission, she had been in remission for three years now and was doing really well, I looked forward to seeing her as she had not been for a few months.

There was another name after her that gave me a bit of a jolt, why on earth had I booked this person in, the last time he came, which was about six months ago, he made several rude and sexist remarks and I swore that I would never treat him again.

I must have been away with the fairies to take the booking, oh well cannot do much about it now but if he gives me any trouble this time man is he going to know about it.

After checking the rest of the bookings I went off to the living-room to watch a horror movie on TV nothing like a good horror movie to relax one.

Monday morning came around fast and furious, it was mainly straight forward massage clients, with one needing Acupressure for her sciatic nerve. All in all a pleasant day.

It was not until my second last client of the day that I had premonition that something was not quite right. Halfway through the massage my client mentioned that she had been talking to Melanie East at church last Sunday and Melanie let slip that she had to see her doctor on Monday (today) as he had phoned her on Friday with the result of her latest test results.

From what Mrs. Claire was saying it did not sound like good news, I hoped that she was wrong. I would have to wait and see what happened tomorrow when Melanie was due for her appointment.

Whilst I was cleaning up and waiting for my last client of the day the phone rang, deciding to answer it. It turned out to be my ex-boyfriend saying he was sorry about Valentine's Day and would I like to go out to dinner on Thursday night, mind you this is only about three months after Valentine's Day.

I told him that apart from the fact that he was in fact several months too late with an apology I already had plans for Thursday night (not an untruth, Jack and I had plans for take away again, well I did Jack would have his usual dog food).

The ex then said what about Friday night then, what is it about some people that they just do not get it, NO I have a date get the message, bye!!

By this time I was seething, pity my last client just as well he is the strong silent type, all though that could change after this next massage.

When I look back on my years as a Remedial Massage Therapist I think how funny and strange it was that I got into it.

I was working in Adult Education at the time and had developed a bad headache which progressively got worse as the day wore on, by late afternoon I had to leave work. One of my students mentioned that there was 'this guy who does massage and he is pretty good, he is pretty good and he could help you'.

By this time I would have asked the Devil himself for help, anyway I got the name and phone number of the guy off my student, and before leaving phoned him up.

As it turned out he only lived a few doors up from where I was living, talk about a small world.

I told him that I had a very bad headache bordering on a migraine, he said to come around now as he had a spot vacant.

When I walked into the house I began to wonder if I had done the right thing. I was shown into the kitchen and asked to wait.

A short time later a woman emerged from along the hall followed by a man, turned out the woman was a client and the man was the masseur.

He introduced himself and asked me to follow him into the other room please, I was shown into a very small room at the front of the house which was somewhat crowded with a large massage table, chair cupboard and small table.

Numerous charts of point of massage adorned the walls.

I was asked to sit down then Errol (Errol Clark was his name) then proceeded to ask me a bit about myself and my medical history when that was done he asked me to undress then hop up on the table.

From the moment he touched my back I knew that I had made the right decision, not only was he the best massage therapist I have ever come across he turned out to be a very good friend.

It is strange how things change in our life, during the massage he got to talking about how busy he was and that he had been trying to find someone to train but to date had no success.

I jokingly said that maybe I could do it, he did not say anything but when the massage was finished he asked to see my hands, I thought he was just checking to see if anything was wrong with them.

It turned out that he wanted to see how strong my hands were.

As I was leaving he asked me if I could come back to see him in two days' time, I said yes thinking that it would be a follow-up massage on today's treatment.

Well to cut a long story short, I went back two days later, the headache had cleared up and I was feeling better than I had for a long time.

I again was sitting waiting in the kitchen, it would have been about twenty minutes later that Errol came out of his room and asked me to follow him.

I got quite a surprise when I entered to see a man lying face down on the table.

Errol turned to me and said, "Would you massage this gentleman's shoulders for me, I'll show you what I mean then you can do it."

Ok maybe my joking about being a masseur might be serious after all.

I did the massage as I was shown and after about fifteen minutes Errol said that was fine and would I mind waiting again till he finished as he would like to talk to me.

The outcome of all this was that I agreed to train as a massage therapist under his supervision, it was not until many years later and several Massage Certificates later, that I thank my lucky stars that I had the opportunity to train under the best massage person ever, he taught me so much and started me on a path that I have enjoyed also.

Over the years I have caught up with Errol a couple of times, he divorced and re-married and moved with his new wife up to the hills where they have a small B&B and he continues to massage to the best of my knowledge to this day.

It is funny now thinking back over my eighteen years of massage I do wonder how I survived the first few years when I was so 'raw' and new to the whole business. I do know that if it was not for Errol I would never have done so.

CHAPTER FIVE

Back in the 60's Prostitution could not be 'advertised' as such so 'Massage Parlours" became the by-word of the sex trade.

Unfortunately even today it still leaves its mark and saying you are a Massage Therapist at times still has to be explained.

You could be out at a party or some other gathering and there would always be the inevitable question, "What sort of work do you do?"

Well as soon as you answered Massage Therapist you could see the eyes glaze over and then the person would look you up and down, the tone of the voice then changed to either one of disgust or one of 'interest' depending on the sex of the person you were talking to.

Yes they were thinking along the wrong track, talk about one track minds.

I remember one woman actually asking me did I ever perform any 'unusual sex requests', I told her I was a genuine Massage Therapist and NOT a sex worker and suggested that she look up the word Therapist in relation to massage, I am sure to this day that she still thinks I am a 'lady of the night.'

As I mentioned earlier I have had my fair share of calls from guys who thought the same thing. The first call I ever received made me really upset to think that anyone could think such a thing boy how naïve I was then, not that I did get many phone calls because people in general are much better educated and now I can sally forth with a cutting remark, now that is progress.

You know Kings Cross in Sydney, Australia, is the mecca for prostitution, transvestites and other assorted sex workers. Back in the 60's it used to be a fun place to visit, pro's stood around outside the buildings soliciting customers and nearly all the sex workers were over 21 – it was the place to go to have a 'gander' at what life was like.

Now it has all changed, the last time I was there most of the girls on the game are very young, and most are drugged out of their minds.

There was one really beautiful young girl standing outside one of the sleazy cheap hotels soliciting, I got talking to her and asked her why she was doing it, as she could have been a model or something.

She took one look at me and said she got into it for the money and for fun and now it is too late, booze, drugs and her pimp make sure she can't leave.

She was drinking out of a paper cup which turned out to be Vodka the only way she could get through a night as some of her customers require 'special' sex – anything involving S&M to anal was the go, I have never felt more sad for a human being in my whole life, what a waste of a beautiful young girl.

I have never been back to Kings Cross and have no wish to ever go back again, things have changed and not for the better.

I suppose looking back that over the years I I have been lucky that I only really had two bad experiences with massage.

The first was just a few months into my new practice. I had set up in the back of a shop in town and you had to go to the rear to enter.

A guy phoned one Saturday morning, it was fairly late in the morning, saying he had pulled a muscle in his back and was in pain. I arranged for him to meet me at the clinic at 2.00pm.

When he arrived I noticed that he seemed to be walking ok, now that should have told me something, but being fairly new to massage I ignored it.

Anyway I lead him into the clinic and proceeded to take down all his details, his name and address should also have warned me.

I finished up and asked him to undress down to his jocks and leave him, five minutes later I return he is sitting on the edge of the table in his jocks, I ask him to lie on his stomach.

I start to massage, I ask him where he has the most pain, he says in his groin, now I start to get a funny feeling about this.

I should mention that as it is a week-end I am in the clinic on my own, my receptionist does not work on Saturdays (I have not had a receptionist for some time now as working from home I do not need one it also saves a heap of money).

Anyhow I ask him why he said his back hurt when he phoned, he said that if he did not have a problem he would not have got an appointment. By now I was starting to feel quite alarmed, asking him just what his problem was, he stated bluntly that the felt like a cheap fuck and so here he was, if he called a pro in the town he lived in his wife would find out, beside I was fairly cheap (I charged $50 an hour back then) and a pro would cost double that.

I stepped back from the tale and told him he had three minutes to get his clothes on and leave, he laughed and started to get off the table, "Hey come on just a quickie will do, so long as you make it a good fuck."

I moved to the front door and screamed, I reckon that he must have been doing his pants up as he flew out the door, luckily the couple who lived next door to the shop were just going out of their place and heard me scream.

Both came running, the jerk by now was in his car and heading off down the road.

I collapsed on the door step and started to cry, my rescuers became very concerned, I explained what had happened, I can still remember them being very angry on my behalf and then they took charge and lead me back into the clinic and sat me in a chair.

They asked if I wanted to phone the police, I declined as there was nothing that could be done really.

I learned my lesson that day and now whenever I have a sixth sense about a potential client I err on the side of caution, a massage therapist's life is not all gloss and glamour.

The second time was some years later I had a new client who had come in for relief of lower back pain injury. All was going well, when I felt something on my leg, I ignored it thinking I had just brushed against the table, a few minutes later I felt it again no mistaking what it was this time.

My client had grabbed my leg, again I ignored it thinking he has just made an involuntary move on his part.

Well a few minutes later all that went out the window as he grabbed me on the crotch, I yelled, he jumped up and swore, I asked him what the hell he was doing, his comment, "Just grabbing a feel."

Instead of telling him to get the hell out I sweetly told him to please get back on the table face down, now anyone who knows me would know that if I started talking 'nicely' to someone who had offended me they would be very smart to run.

You know it is funny but after the massage he never came back again, people have told me I have very strong hands, guess he just could not take a 'strong handed' massage anymore.

Over the years I have treated many and varied injuries and ailments and seen many and varied clients, there are many that stick in my mind but one in particular comes to mind.

It was about mid-way in my career when I had a phone call from an elderly gentleman (and he was a gentleman), he said he was having trouble with leg pains and was finding it hard to sleep.

My first thought was sciatic pain, I made an appointment for him for two days hence. The day of the appointment arrived and my new client with it.

Mr. Weir turned out to be a man in his late 70's, he had been widowed for the past three years – he seemed fit and well but did walk with a slight limp.

After taking all his particulars I asked him to undress and get on the massage table face down and that I would be back in five minutes.

I came back in and began the massage I had been right it was a sciatic problem, after explaining that I would be using Acupressure combined with the massage and it could be a bit painful but would help the problem he seemed ok with it.

As we were talking during the massage he mentioned how lonely he was after his wife's death, they had no children and most of his friends were either in homes or had passed on.

He said that he had enjoyed a full and joyful life with his wife and missed that, he was quiet for a minute then asked, "Do you do relief massage?"

It took me a minute to work out what he wanted, he was asking if I in fact did 'hand jobs' for sexual relief. You know for the first time in my life I was actually sorry that I did not do so, professionalism and standards held fast and I had to politely tell him no, I did not.

That this gentleman had to ask such a thing must have been so hard for him and even harder for me, sometimes life can be the pits.

Anyway back to here and now, it was the day of Melanie East's appointment, I had a fairly busy morning and had to fit in a new client that day as she was in pain from a pulled neck muscle.

I had only just finished cleaning up from the last client when Melanie arrived, she was very quiet which was unusual for her, getting her settled on the table I got out the special oil that I use on clients such as Melanie (these are essential oils mixed with Olive Oil which is what I prefer to mix my essential oils with, this one was Lavender as Melanie preferred it and it does have a soothing effect).

I don't do my usual remedial massage on Melanie it is more of a relaxation one – and hardly any pressure is used expect on her neck and shoulders where she hold a lot of tension.

I chatted about nothing in particular giving Melanie a chance to relax, she did not say anything for a while then said that she had been called back to the doctors the other day, the cancer was back and this time it was very aggressive.

At a time like this one does not answer with the usual platitudes I simply asked her what the prognosis was and could I do anything to help.

She said that the doctor had said that she could have two years at the most and that this time there was nothing that could be done.

I did not reply, there was nothing to say, we finished the massage and I said that if at any time she needed help with the pain management or stress to just give me a call I would fit her in no matter what time.

I gave her a hug and with that she got dressed, paid and left.

I saw her only twice after that, it was only six months later that she passed away leaving her distraught husband and two wonderful children, sometimes I wonder what the Gods are thinking.

I have had a lot of elderly clients over the years and many have passed on, none have affected me like Melanie's death.

I can honestly say that she was one of the nicest people I have ever had the privilege of knowing.

CHAPTER SIX

Back in the dark dim ages when I first started training under Errol, he 'volunteered' me to help him every Monday (which was my day off) to help him massage one of the local football teams about twenty minutes' drive from where we lived, little did I know what I was letting myself in for.

I got up on the Monday morning and at 8.30am presented myself at Errol's door, we would then drive to the town where each week Errol had the use of a vacant shop.

We would proceed to set up two massage tables and at precisely 9.30am the first of the footy boys would arrive.

Now I being very innocent at that time thought that we would be massaging about 8 footballers at the most, turns out that we actually had over 14 to massage plus a few 'extras' and a few locals thrown in.

So we start working away, about four hours later we take a short break for a cup of tea and something to eat. What I learnt from that experience is that a cold cup of tea and an overripe banana can keep you going for most of the day!

Well we went hard at it once again till around 7.00p when we again had another break, me being me had thought that we would be knocking off about now (if not long before this) no such luck.

Anyway I was sent across the road to pick up fish and chips for tea, I get back to a lukewarm cup of tea and find four young men already waiting, cold fish and chips got to be the order of the day for the rest of the footy season.

We finally finish about midnight, packing up I was so exhausted I could have wept. In the car on the way home Errol casually mentions that we have a client to see on the way home, a farmer, he had hurt his lower lumbar.

I said wasn't it a bit late for another client and wouldn't he be in bed?

Errol assured me that it was fine to be calling in at nearly 1.00am in the morning, the farmer would be up and waiting for us, sure enough he was right oh the joys of massage!

Well finally we got back home about 3.00am, then I only had a couple of hours sleep before getting up and going to work at my regular job which at time was a Training and Development Officer with SkillShare, long since closed down.

I did complete the rest of the football season with Errol and learned things that I would never had learn out of any text book, plus I got to meet some charming, funny and down to earth young men, all of whom were appreciative of the massage and the time devoted to keeping them fit.

It was funny how at first they were shy of getting undressed in front of a female, I mean being strong virile young men one would have thought that they would think nothing of it, not so.

But after the first few times they then just laughed, stripped down and got onto the table, and believe me you had no time to wonder or admire any of them you were far too busy.

Just think all those near naked young men and me with no time to perve, there is no justice in the world.

I got to know quite a few of the boys over the time I was massaging, they were all passionate about football and had funny, sad and at times irrelevant stories to tell about it.

I remember mentioning to one of the young men that I was having trouble getting a fire grate as they were hard to get hold of.

Well the next week he turned up with a hand-made grate that he had gotten one of his mates to make for me, he would not accept any payment from me said it was his way of saying thanks for all the effort I put in.

Well life goes on and I eventually moved away and only saw Errol once after that which was at his second marriage.

As I said earlier he is still massaging and no matter what anyone says he is still the best massage therapist that I have ever come across.

I remember that during the time I was working with Errol I occasionally got to take his place if he was called away or something.

One night I had not long gotten home from work when the phone rang, it was Errol could I do a massage for him later that night as he had to go to a unscheduled meeting (he was head of the St. John's Ambulance Corp) said yes that would be no problem.

Well down I went to his place about 7.45pm and checking that all was set up in the massage room waited for his client.

At 10 past 8.00 in she comes, "Who are you, where is Errol?"

I told her that I was taking Errol's place as had been inadvertently called away, you know this is the first time that I have actually seen someone's face turn purple.

"What do you mean *you* are going to do the massage, I want Errol, I don't want you!"

Try as I might I could not pacify her, in the end she stormed out and said she would talk to Errol about this. 'This' presumably was me, no problem I left a note and went back home to have some tea and a glass of wine.

It was not until the next night that I got a phone call from Errol, he had seen the funny side of it, which was more than I did at the time.

"Sorry I forgot it was Lorraine, she only likes a man to massage her."

Now I could have made a really cheeky comeback at that, but declined I mean what could one state but the obvious, that it 'must be the only time a man would want to put his hands on her, as most would run a mile', not saying she is ugly or anything but I have seen better looking toads than her.

It has just struck me that there must be a lot of you who have never had a massage and have no idea what goes on, for the uninitiated here goes!

Let us assume you are a new client, you come into the clinic, and first thing you see is the massage table. This is usually a very strong padded vinyl affair, mine has arm rests and a separate head rest along with vinyl cushions to put under your knees or ankles if required.

This is all supported on a very strong metal frame which is made to support a fairly heavy person.

Ok so you now sit down and I proceed to fill in your new client form, which includes your name, address etc, then I proceed to get all your relevant medical history and anything that might affect a massage.

For instance, if you have a heart condition I would need a letter from your doctor saying that you would benefit from a massage.

If you have a pacemaker then it is a definite no to massage, that also goes for any infectious conditions such as shingles, with everything clear I explain what treatment you will get.

Massage is usually a full-body one, that means that I work on you from head to toe back and front.

If you are a female I ask if you want your breasts massaged as some people do not like this done, there is nothing sexual about it, it is simply part of the massage and I do not massage directly over the breast but around.

If you are a male do not even think about asking if your penis gets a massage, it might but I can assure you would NOT like it!

Ok you are on the table face down, I start to work on your back, long firm strokes down your back on either side of your spine, then work back up along your side. This is repeated several times, then I usually progress to the shoulders, arms, then buttocks, legs and feet, then back to your neck and massage that down both sides if necessary I would apply Acupressure to any points requiring it, Acupressure is the use of fingers or thumbs on specific pressure points in the body to relieve the pressure on areas of pain as in the sciatic nerve.

It is exactly the same as Acupuncture except there are no needles used – same pressure points.

Then you get turned over (bit like basting isn't it) well now you are lying on your back, comfy?

I proceed to massage your chest, abdomen, legs and feet and then back up to your arms and hands I finish off with a neck massage, which is drawing and pulling up towards me (I am standing behind your head) then a nice scalp massage, by now you are feeling quite relaxed or it has been a remedial massage, which involves a lot more pressure and more stretching and pulling where required, then maybe quite sore.

Now you slither off the table, get dressed, pay me – most important and make another appointment, then glide out the door, well that wasn't so bad was it?

I must admit that remedial massage is a bit more involved than that as it involves working on a particular area to relieve pain and can be quite painful in itself but the results are that in the end you feel better, which is what massage is all about, making the client well.

I will never forget the first time I had to sit for my very first massage certificates. It was at a local hall and the examiner/teacher had set up twelve tables around the hall. There were both male and female present, now I remember at this time I was naively innocent in the ways of massage and thought it would be separate rooms for the sexes, yes well that was my first mistake.

Well the examiner proceeds to tell us to take off our shoes and stretch (we are all wearing loose comfortable clothing) well off come the shoes and I start stretching, next we are asked to stretch to the sky then to the floor, sure I can do this (mind you I would have trouble stretching to the floor now I think).

Then we have to stand with our legs apart and stretch out and touch the person next to you, hang on, am I in the right room?

Anyway we stretch and as things progress the examiner takes us through the basic techniques of massage, asking questions of each of us as she goes, by this time the morning has flown by and it is time for lunch.

Putting my shoes back on I wonder out to the kitchen and get my sandwiches out of the fridge and make a cup of coffee, everyone is fairly relaxed at this stage and we laugh and joke among ourselves.

Lunch over we go back into the room ok now this is where it gets interesting, we are asked to pair up, so female to female, male to male, right, wrong try other way round male/female, ok this is fun, then comes the axe, we are asked to strip and one of us get on the massage table (the one doing the massage does get to keep their clothes on at this stage).

We are asked to do a complete massage, I am lucky (or not) to be the first on the table, after trying to get undressed so that no-one can see me, which in a large hall with no nooks or crannies was a lost cause to start with, looking back and realize how stupid it was as no one was interested in anyone else just trying to remember the correct points of massage.

Well the massage starts and when the examiner gets to us she stands there for a while watching then asks my 'partner' relevant questions. He appears to answer them ok and then she goes off to someone else.

Massage completed we change places and I begin the massage, the examiner comes back and I am sure she hates me as she manages to ask me nearly every question that is NOT in the book, by this time I am wondering if a change in career would be on the cards, anyway I complete the massage and my partner climbs off the table and gets dressed.

We are then asked to assemble in a circle around the examiner and sit. Feels like kindergarten ok we sit, she proceeds to tell us that we have all done an excellent job and that there were one or two who would make excellent masseurs, and guess what I was one of them. Someone up there likes me.

Looking back those first certificates were the hardest out of all the years that I studied. Seems silly now when I think about it, but we were really put through our paces that day I often wonder out of all those in the room how many continued to practice.

I mentioned earlier that I had a client booked in who was prone to sexist comments and was a real pain in the ass type and I could not understand why I had booked him in.

Anyway the day of his appointment came and he arrived, late as previous, and bombastic as well.

Well he had hardly sat down when he started on his opinion of females that most of them were useless, etc, WRONG!

Now I am not one to say anything (well not usually anyway) as the client is always right but this was too much so I let him have it both barrels. The upshot was dead silence in the room, well there goes a client, how wrong I was.

He actually apologized and actually smiled, turns out every one is scared of him and just lets him get away with it, I was one of only two people that had ever stood up to him, and gained his respect from that day forward.

Strange as it may seem he is still a person I call my friend to this day, you just never know what will happen if you have the guts to stand up for what you believe in, you just might find a new friend and supporter, or worst case loose a client that was not worth it anyway.

CHAPTER SEVEN

There is no denying that 9/11 changed the world and the way we think and live, this was brought home to me in a very strange way.

It was a Sunday morning I was just thinking about doing some work on the house when the phone rang.

The man on the other end said that he was passing through and had managed to pull a muscle in his shoulder he was in a fair amount of pain and had gotten my name out of the phone book and would he be able to come in for a massage.

Hoping to discourage him I mentioned the fee for an out of hours appointment, he surprised me by saying that was fine. So I told him where I lived and went and got the clinic ready.

A short time later a rather expensive grey car pulled up at the front door and out got a dark skinned slim man.

I noticed that he was barefoot and he had one arm slightly bent, he appeared to be walking slightly bent over also.

In he came and as was customary I asked for all his details, he said was that really necessary as he was just passing through and would not be back again.

He seemed to be somewhat put out by my asking so for once I decided to forgo all the usual paperwork and asked him to undress and get on the table.

Once he was on the table I asked him where he felt the most pain, he said in his right shoulder on feeling around the shoulder there appeared to be a 'knot' in it, I checked his left shoulder also and noted that his left arm was bent and was shorter than his right.

I made a comment about it and he said that he had been born with a slightly deformed left arm but that it did not worry him.

As I was working on his back I asked him if he was on holiday here, he said no he was just down from Sydney for a couple of days rest from work. I asked him what sort of work he did.

Now this is where it gets interesting, first the guy gets out of his expensive car in bare feet, he does not want to answer any questions about himself and guess what his job was.

He said that he was a surgeon in one of the large hospitals in Sydney and just wanted to get away for some R&R.

Ok me being me, the first thing I wanted to know was if he was a surgeon how did he manage to operate with a bung arm?

So, I asked him. His answer well he did not have to life his arm up to do surgery so he managed fine.

Ok that was logical, NOT.   Warning bells started going off in my head so I kept asking questions.

Had he enjoyed his stay here, when was he heading back, did he like Sydney, had he been working in the hospital for very long, and wasn't the Opera House amazing.

He said he had only been in the area for a few days and liked what he had seen, he was heading back the next day and yes he liked Sydney and he had not been to the Opera House yet but liked the photos he had seen and he said he had been here for two years.

I let it lie for the time being and concentrated on working the stiffness out of his joints.

As he was starting to relax he asked me a strange question.

He said he had driven past the police station on his way here (which in fact is not on the way but a round a bout way of getting here) and noticed that there was no-one on duty, is that normal for here?

Weird, I said that we had a small contingent of police here but there was a large police force between the towns round a bout and could be called on if need be.

I jokingly said was he planning a bank robbery or something.

He laughed and said no, no bank robbery.

As I was nearing the end of the hour, he asked if I could continue for another hour as he was just starting to feel better, ok his money and it was fine by me.

So I continued with the massage and worked over the whole body once again.

As I was completing the massage he asked me how far it was to Wagga Wagga from here, now that is a strange question as if he as he said he was heading back to Sydney, Wagga was the other way.

I told him about an hour and a half drive and left it at that.

When the massage was finished he got dressed, paid me the money for the two hours, thanked me and left.

Now I do not stereotype anyone but there was something about this guy that had me on edge.

He was not an Australian, he was slight of build, dark in appearance of Arabic descent, drives a flash car, has a bung arm yet says he is a surgeon, was heading back to Sydney yet wanted to go via Wagga Wagga, did not want to answer personal questions, and had a wad of cash in his wallet, yes I did notice that.

Anyway he was gone and that was the last of it.

Only it did not turn out that way.

Next day I was about to sit down to have a bite of lunch before starting work again when the phone rang, it was this same man again, he wanted to see if he could come in for a massage later that day.

I could not help myself but blurted out, "Oh, I thought you were back in Sydney today?"

He said that he was taking an extra day and felt that another massage would benefit him before heading back.

I told him that I was sorry but I was fully booked.

He said it did not matter if it was later he would pay the out of hours fee.

The answer was still no, I did not want to massage that guy ever **again**.

It was not until the following week that someone asked me had I heard about the attempted supposed terrorist attack on the Army Base at Wagga Wagga last week.

It turned out that three men attempted to enter the Army Base there with the intention of blowing some of it up.

They were interrupted and all three escaped the police were still trying to find them.

Seems that someone at the base had spotted the intruders and given the alarm, an explosive device was found but there was still no sign of the three men.

They were described as medium build, with dark complexions around 30 – 40 years of age, they were considered dangerous.

To this day I wonder if the man that came for the massage that day was one of the three men it all seemed to fit, guess I will never know, and no I did not mention to the police, I really had nothing to offer but a gut feeling and where would I have told them to look, yes I had the colour of the car but did not think to get a make or model or number plate.

We think it will never happen to us or happen here, we just never know.

CHAPTER EIGHT

Now usually when a new client comes and I have gone over everything and taken down all their particulars, I make a point of telling them to undress down to their (depends on sex) knickers or underpants.

Well for some reason either on this particular day I had a mind freeze or the new client did not hear me.

I left him to get undressed and when I came back five minutes later there he is, face down on the table and a bare backside shining up at me.

(Thank god it was face down)

So very nonchalantly I grab a towel and drape it over his posterior, half an hour later after finishing his back I ask him to turn over, being VERY careful to hold the towel in a strategic place as he turns.

Needless to say as soon as the massage was finished I departed the room quickly to allow him to dress.

One thing I forgot to tell you a Massage Therapist is not only a therapist, but doctor, physiatrist, marriage counsellor, advice to the love-lorn and whatever else comes around, bit like a hairdresser, we know all and tell nothing (well until many years later that is).

Mind you sometimes the things you get told would make your hair stand on end, now recently I had a young man (anyone under 40 is young to me) he had been coming for quite a while and at first you could not get a word out of him, it made for a very long and quiet massage as people usually like to chat and the time goes faster.

Anyway this day he hopped on the table as usual and said his usual 'hi' which is about all I usually get out of him.

Well he must have decided that I was someone he could open up to, either that or he was at his wits end.

Seems that he has his eye on a particular lady and being somewhat shy he did not know how to approach her (I might add that he still lived with his mummy and yes he was in his late 30's)

Yes, now you get the picture, anyway he starts to tell me that this woman is everything that he could ever want in a woman, now where have I heard that before.

He is sure that mummy would approve – told you – now the first thing I think is how on earth does he know what she is like if he has never spoken to her, for all he knows she could be a mass murderer or something, so me being the sweet, kind, thoughtful....ok back to reality.

I ask him, turns out he had said 'Hi' to her and she had smiled at him (yes well I do that all the time, now I know what men are thinking I had better stop smiling).

Anyway to cut to the chase he is desperate to ask her out, so here I jump in with my two cents worth and tell him next time he sees her, say 'hello' and try and get her chatting then he can ask her if she is seeing anyone and if she says no, ask her out, simple really.

Well my erstwhile Casanova agrees to this and thanking me trips out of the clinic with the prospect of waltzing down the aisle with his beloved.

Well some weeks later he returns for his usual massage and seems extremely happy. Turns out he did manage to speak to her and as luck would have it she fancied him) Now to put the record straight he is quite a good looking guy for all that) anyway the upshot was that by now they had been on two date and he was taking her to meet mummy for dinner that Sunday (well this could be the end of a beautiful relationship, I have actually met mummy, not my cup of tea but each to his own).

I forgot all about him and did not see him again for a couple of months.

When he did come back for another massage he seemed very downcast, seems that mummy dearest did not take to the new girlfriend, and he can't desert mummy now can he.

Yes I know what you are thinking I put my bit foot in it and said dump mummy dearest, well actually I didn't, I actually said that maybe he should be making his own decisions at his age and if he really liked the woman then maybe he should pursue it.

Yes you guessed it one less client, gee some people are hard to please.

I have had many strange and funny things happen over the years and one incident stands out in my mind.

I had booked a new client, he arrived and after the usual preliminaries got down to massaging. I asked him what his main problem was, he said that he really did not have any problems he just wanted a massage.

Ok moving on, now you would think that I would have learned by now that when someone starts off that they do not have any problems then start asking me question I would smell a rat, not always the case.

He started off asking me if I had a partner, no, did I like living alone, yes it's ok, did I go out much, depends on how much you classify as 'out much' – I wonder does a trip to the pizza shop count? He continued, did I like living here etc, anyway I thought nothing o it, just a new client being curious, WRONG!

As it turned out I got a phone call two days later from this same client, the only reason he came for a massage was to 'check me out', then he proceeded to ask me out.

Rule number one – I do not go out with clients, rule number two – no one 'checks me out', rule number three – tell soon to be ex-client he can go jump.

Now if he had been nice about the whole thing I might have considered breaking rule number one, hell I might have considered breaking all of them.

But I mean the cheek of the man – 'checking me out' just like I was a piece of meat on a slab, no thanks.

As it turned out he said that a mate of his had mentioned that I was single and he thought that by getting a massage he would be one up and get a date.

Sure in what dimension.

Looking back he has been the only client that has ever asked me out, most clients (the male variety we are talking about here) come to get a specific problem fixed and by the time I have finished working on them they have just about enough energy to crawl out the door, the last thing on their minds would be asking me out.

Which all things considered is a pity sometimes as I do get some really nice guys but no, rules are rules.

CHAPTER NINE

You know looking back it does not seem possible that I have been working as a Remedial Massage Therapist for the past eighteen years.

At first it started out as just a way to earn some extra money whilst working my full-time job.

Well the part-time massage job soon turned into a full-time flat out job, I could not say when the transition took place, probably one day when I decided that I had enough of working for someone else (at the time I was Managing a Credit Union but had become more and more disillusioned with the job).

Looking back it seemed to be only a few days that after deciding that enough was enough I chucked in my job and throwing caution to the wind ordered a massage table and all the trimmings, plus oil and another table top massage for neck and shoulders only.

I went out and ordered a sign to go on the front fence, then went a brought new towels, green polo shirts and white shorts for me and then back home to re-arrange the small front bedroom into a clinic.

It was a couple of days later that I started to shake and wonder what the hell I had done. I had left a well-paying job and now I had no income, no fallback plan, just the knowledge that from now on I had to make my own living my way, I would either sink or swim.

Well not only did I survive but survived very well right from the moment (well not quite) that the sign went up on the front fence people started to dribble in.

Initially I had put a few advertisements in the local paper and also lashed out with the last of my cash to put coasters in one of the local clubs (this proved to be a costly mistake as I never did get anyone from the club come for a massage).

Before long word had gotten around and from then on I never looked back, I was a success!

Well to be honest it took a lot of hard work and at times, stretching my rules about what hours I would work as being new to the game, not the OTHER game not the game you are thinking.

I wound up falling into the trap of taking clients when they wanted to come and was working all hours.

This soon changed and they came when I wanted them to – ok so I did make exceptions to this but only if it was an emergency or I know that they could only come after hours, see I am nice.

I did initially do home visits but soon learned that this was not a good idea.

The last home visit I did was after a gentleman phoned and asked if I could do a home visit to his elderly mother as she was unable to get out of the house due to her advanced age and also she was crippled with arthritis.

I arranged to make the house call on the following Thursday night at 6.00pm as this was the only time I could fit the visit in and suited the client.

Well I get to the address given and ring the bell, a gentleman answers the door, he would be in this late 50's and says to come in, he shows me where to set up my table (I have a portable massage table) and then says that he will get his mother she is lying down, he won't be long.

Well I set up the table and when after fifteen minutes the mother still has not appeared I start to worry.

Is she dead and he is too scared to tell me, has she decided that she does not want a massage after all, has he gone to China to get her?

Another 10 minutes passes and I am about to pack up and leave when in walks 'mother', it is the gentleman that opened the door and the same guy that booked the massage for her, only it is not a little old lady that entered but the guy himself, only he is dressed in a grey wig, his face is powdered up to within an inch of its life and is complete with bright spots of rouge, red lips and blue eye shadow, he/she is dressed – sorry not dressed – in a corset, suspenders and thick Lyle stockings, a padded bra with a cardigan over her/his shoulders.

All I can do is stare, WTF is going on here?
He/she proceeds to say that 'she' has been looking forward to her massage and do I mind if she leaves her clothes on and could she get a shoulder and arm massage please as she has been in so much pain lately.

Ok by now I am thinking how quickly can I pack up this table and run, but hey, I am a professional and I can handle this.

So I sit her on the table and proceed to massage her neck, shoulders and arms. Thirty five minutes later I tell her she can get down now and perhaps she would like to get dressed.

Well she leaves the room and I sit down and try not to laugh, now I know why 'mother' could not come into the clinic, to this day I am still not sure whether he/she did this thing on a regular basis, needless to say I never visited again.

But he did pay me and gave me a tip for being so good with the massage.

You know if the same thing happened today I would probably accept it as normal, after all these years I have found that I can handle just about anything and that very little surprises me now.   How things change.

Funny but the clients I love best are the elderly they hardly ever complain even when they are in so much pain that anyone else would be screaming up the walls, they are nearly all easy to work on and I do get a great delight in helping to relieve their pain, even if only for a short while.

However there is always one exception to the rule, and this would have to be Mable Brown, she comes in once a month for a massage.

I have considered paying another therapist to take her, only thing is when I did mention it to one therapist she not only told me to go and do something that would be anatomically impossible but painful to myself as well.

Anyway today is 'Mable Day' or as I call it take a grip on yourself and don't swear day.

Mable is one of those people who no matter what happens to them they would find something to complain about, if she won Lotto she would complain that she would now have her pension taken off her.

I really dread this day but do not have the courage to tell her not to come again (yes I know I am a wimp) so here it is Mabel arrives and then proceeds to tell me that the clinic is too cold, now I am sweating and the room could cook eggs it is that hot.

So I open the window to cool it down for her, not good enough do I want her to catch a chill, ok so I close the window wishing her head was under it and grit my teeth.

I leave her to get undressed (I do have some elderly clients that I help to undressed and dressed) Mable is one person that I would not even consider offering to help as I am sure that I would probably strangle her with her stockings.

Anyway five minutes later I come back into the clinic, Mabel is sitting on the table wrapped in a large towel, which I may add is wrapped around her tighter than a mummies bandages.

Well she lies down on the table and I proceed to try and get the towel from around her so that I can work on her back, after practically turning myself inside out I get it loosened enough so that I can work on her.

I am massaging her back, not nearly as hard as I would like to, when she proceeds to tell me that my hands are cold, ok I warm them up and get back to it. I am pressing too hard do I want to bruise her, only round her throat.

After ten minutes she then proceeds to tell me that she doesn't know why she comes here for a massage as she is so sore after, surely she should not be sore and why don't I put a coffee machine in the clinic so that people can at least have a cup of coffee after their massage.

She is sure that more people would come and make use of the facilities. Facilities? Massage or coffee club? I resist the urge to tell her that this is not a five star resort, just one very tired massage therapist working on one pain in the ass client and if she is not careful she will be getting a 'hard handed' massage that would do her the world of good, and she would then really have something to complain about.

I take a deep breath and continue getting down to her arms I proceed to work down to her hands and massage them (she does have arthritis in her hands and the massage helps) but it is a stronger massage here than anywhere else to help relieve the pain and get deeper into the tissue.

So here we go, wait for it, "Oh you are hurting me, why do you press so hard, my poor hands you are so cruel, really I won't come here anymore".

Really, there is a god after all...hooray.

Well massage finished I leave her to get dressed, coming back in after a few minutes she is putting on her coat, "Well I really enjoyed that dear, same time next month then?"

Why oh why do I bother and here I thought she was finally giving up. I book her in and then sit down and put my head in my hands and, if it was not for the next client would have cried, or screamed and thrown something.

I suppose I should be grateful for her, she obviously likes coming here and I think I am probably the only person in the whole town who has not told her where to go, see being professional has it, now not sure whether it is compensations or commiserations.

CHAPTER TEN

Now for those purists amongst you who are just dying to know where massage all started I will endeavor to enlighten you.

The earliest records of massage were found on wall paintings on ancient Egyptian tombs at around 2500 BC, they depict individuals receiving a massage (or kneading as it was recorded) there are also records in China of massage being used around 3000 BC.

In India around the same time the art of massage (Ayurveda) was performed.

Records show that in Ancient Greece the athletes were given massage to keep them at peak condition, Ancient Rome also used massage, in all it was found that massage could reduce stress produce a deep relaxation and help reduce injuries, off of which continue today.

Massage is not something new it has been around for centuries. It was in the 60's that massage came into contact with prostitution (as mentioned earlier) and then anyone doing 'massage' was labelled as a 'lady of the night'.

It has taken quite a few years for it to now be accepted as a legitimate healing process and not a 'red light proposition' (although even in this day and age some people need to be enlightened on the subject.)

To be a masseur you need to be fit, healthy, dedicated to wanting to promote health and well-being in clients, prepared to study and study hard to obtain your qualifications, have a thick skin, this I would consider the prime objective of any massage therapist, must have a sense of humour, because you are really going to need it someday.

Strong hands are a must and not just for strangling some clients no matter how much you would like to, patience (yes I now I lack that, but can you honestly blame me after what I have told you).

And last but not least, respect for yourself and your clients, if you do respect yourself it would be all too easy to go 'by the wayside' and indeed put us all back into the 60's definition of massage once again.

We still have to fight against this every time you pick up a newspaper under 'adult relationships' is, yes you guessed it, 'massage' the old red herring is back and bright as ever and staring us in the face, damn hard to win these day, all we do is but try to enlighten the faint hearted that we are indeed dedicated to looking after their bodies.

NO not sex, will you please get your mind up out of the gutter, I ask you!!

A Massage Therapist is dedicated to one thing helping clients maintain a happy and healthy lifestyle and a body that is fit and active or as well as it can be with shall we say, regular 'maintenance'.

Ok now that all that rubbish is out of the way, would I go and do it all again, the training, the long hours the endless study and whining clients, the aching back, that is me and the endless round.

Yes, definitely even though at times I have been tried beyond the point of endurance, scared, shocked (yes even me) so tired that I could not even bother to get a drink, now that IS tired.

But through it all I have met some wonderful people and had the ultimate pleasure of knowing that I have helped them to achieve better health and to maintain a lifestyle that is all the thanks that I need. The clients I have had in the most part have been wonderful people and I have enjoyed my choice of work.

The Ancient civilizations were right about massage, when used by a capable and trained massage therapist – massage is indeed a god send.

Just one thing before I finish (well maybe a few more things).

I have only remarked on adults getting massage, sorry forgot to mention that children and babies are among the most delightful, well most of the time, to massage.

Massaging a pregnant mother to be is one of the most wonderful experiences anyone could ever have, not only does it relax the mother but you can feel the baby actually coming close to the surface of the skin and relaxing it is truly amazing.

Now nearly all of the children that I have massaged have been great, but there is always one that is the exception, and that one was the child of one of my most obnoxious clients, yes you get the picture.

The little darling boy was mummies little angle, not the word I would have used to describe him, hell on earth would be more like it.

Mummy brings him into the clinic one Saturday morning for a massage, the little dear would be about six years old at the time, seems Julian has hurt his leg and told mummy that he wanted to the 'massage person' – so in they come.

First thing he does is tell me that he does not like me, ok I am fine with that, not exactly fond of you either darling.

Then he tells me that he does not like being touched, ok this should make for an interesting massage. I finally get him on the table with a lot of bribing, yes I do resort to bribes works wonders, that is why I have a lollie jar, mind you a lot of adults seem to need a 'bribe' too.

Anyway back to dear Julian, mummy is talking to him and I run my hands down his leg, wham, I get a kick out of him, mummy tells him to be a good boy and 'not kick the nice lady'.

I won't tell you what he called me, actually did not know that any six year old would even know that word never mind use it.

Anyway after much struggle on everyone's part I manage to massage his leg, now by this time he has decided that I just might be ok after all and has been asking questions as to why I 'pushed' his leg. I tell him to make him better, now something should have warned me that he was up to something, I finished working on his leg and was lifting him off the table, just as he got off and onto the floor he turned and kicked me hard in the shins.

I swore and this time he looked shocked, now pity mummy there or little Julian would have got a very sore bum out of it as it was mummy just said, "Oh you are a naughty boy Julian, don't do that again."

Yes right as if that will work a good whack on his nether regions would work so much better.

It was with great relief that saw them both off, usually my smaller clients are a joy to work with and I rarely have any trouble and most love to come in for their massage.

I must remember to put a note on his chart to watch out for feet getting on and off the table, that is when I could walk without pain.

I have also had the great joy of working with animals mainly dogs and horses.

And contrary to what people believe they love massage and yes it is different from what I would give to a human but the principal is basically the same.

Even though I am now retired I still have some of Jack's doggy friends that still love their massage and yes so does Master Jack.

As dogs get older it is great that I can work on their muscles and give them relief and hopefully more pain free years into their old age.

Yes Massage is a wonderful profession and one that I would recommend to those that feel the need to follow this path, just watch out for the 'strange ones'.